CHAIR YOGA FOR SENIORS

Transform Your Daily Routine With Chair Yoga Tailored Exercises For Seniors With Gentle Movements For Improved Flexibility, Strength, And Balance Without Leaving Your Chair

CONTENTS

1: Introduction

2: Understanding Chair Yoga

3: Getting Started

4: Basic Chair Yoga Poses

5: Chair Yoga Sequences

6: Breathing Techniques and Meditation

7: Modifications and Adaptations

8: Overcoming Common Challenges

9: Integrating Chair Yoga into Daily Life

10: Personal Stories and Testimonials

11: Conclusion

INTRODUCTION

Welcome to "Chair Yoga for Seniors," a book dedicated to promoting health and well-being among older adults through the gentle yet powerful practice of chair yoga. In our golden years, maintaining physical and mental health becomes increasingly important, and chair yoga offers an accessible and effective means to achieve this goal.

A. Purpose of the Book:

The primary aim of this book is to empower seniors to enhance their health and well-being through chair yoga. This practice is uniquely designed to accommodate the needs and limitations of older adults, making yoga both safe and enjoyable. Whether you are seeking to improve your physical flexibility, boost your balance, or cultivate mental clarity, this book provides the tools and guidance necessary to integrate chair yoga into your daily routine.

B. Promoting Health and Well-being:

Chair yoga is a holistic practice that addresses both physical and mental health. This book will guide you through a series of chair yoga exercises specifically tailored to improve mobility, strengthen muscles, and enhance overall physical function. Moreover, the mindful aspects of yoga will help reduce stress, promote relaxation, and enhance mental clarity, contributing to a better quality of life.

C. Addressing Common Challenges:

Aging brings with it unique physical and mental challenges. Many seniors face issues such as reduced flexibility, balance difficulties, joint pain, and decreased cognitive function. Chair yoga offers a gentle approach to overcoming these obstacles, allowing you to maintain independence and vitality. This book will address these common concerns with targeted exercises and mindful practices designed to support your journey to better health.

D. Why Chair Yoga?

Benefits of Yoga Adapted to a Chair:

Chair yoga is an adaptation of traditional yoga that provides a safe and accessible way to practice yoga, particularly for those with limited mobility or balance issues. By performing yoga poses while seated or using a chair for support, you can enjoy the benefits of yoga without the risk of injury. This makes chair yoga an ideal practice for seniors, ensuring that yoga is inclusive and approachable for everyone.

Health Benefits Specific to Seniors:

Engaging in chair yoga offers numerous health benefits, especially tailored to the needs of seniors. Regular practice can lead to improved flexibility, helping to ease stiffness and increase the range of motion in joints. Enhanced balance from chair yoga can reduce the risk of falls, a common concern for older adults. Additionally, the practice promotes mental clarity and emotional well-being, helping to alleviate symptoms of anxiety and depression.

By incorporating chair yoga into your daily routine, you can experience a significant improvement in your overall health and well-being. This book is here to guide you every step of the way, providing detailed instructions, illustrations, and tips to ensure a safe and effective practice. Let's embark on this journey together towards a healthier, happier, and more balanced life.

UNDERSTANDING CHAIR YOGA

A. What is Chair Yoga?

I. Definition and History of Chair Yoga:

Chair Yoga is a gentle form of yoga that can be done while sitting on a chair or standing while using a chair for support. It is particularly designed for people with limited mobility, balance issues, or those who find traditional yoga poses challenging. The use of the chair allows individuals to perform a variety of yoga poses, breathing exercises, and relaxation techniques, making yoga accessible to a wider audience, including seniors.

The history of Chair Yoga is relatively recent, emerging in the late 20th century as part of the broader adaptation and evolution of yoga to suit various populations. Pioneers like Lakshmi Voelker-Binder, who created the "Chair Yoga" program in 1982, played a significant role in developing and popularizing this practice. She aimed to make yoga accessible to everyone, regardless of their physical condition or age, ensuring that the benefits of yoga could be experienced by all.

II. Differences Between Traditional Yoga and Chair Yoga:

Traditional yoga typically involves performing poses on a yoga mat on the floor, requiring a range of motion, strength, and balance. It often includes standing poses, sitting poses, and even inversions. Chair Yoga, on the other hand, adapts these poses to be performed while seated or using a chair for support. This adaptation allows individuals who might struggle with traditional yoga to participate and benefit from the practice.

Key differences include:

Accessibility: Chair Yoga is designed to be accessible to those with limited mobility, seniors, or those recovering from injuries.

Safety: By using a chair, the risk of falls and injuries is significantly reduced, making it a safer option for individuals with balance issues.

Flexibility of Practice: Chair Yoga can be practiced anywhere, whether at home, in a community center, or even at work, as it does not require much space or specialized equipment.

B. Benefits of Chair Yoga for Seniors:

I. Physical Benefits:

Improved Flexibility:

Chair Yoga helps improve flexibility by gently stretching muscles and joints. Regular practice can lead to increased range of motion, which can make everyday activities easier and reduce the risk of injuries. This is particularly important for seniors, as flexibility tends to decrease with age.

Enhanced Strength:

By engaging in Chair Yoga, seniors can build and maintain muscle strength. Poses are designed to target different muscle groups, helping to improve overall body strength. Stronger muscles support better posture, enhance mobility, and contribute to a higher level of independence.

Better Balance:

Balance is crucial for preventing falls, a common concern for seniors. Chair Yoga includes poses and exercises that focus on balance and stability. Regular practice can enhance proprioception (the sense of self-movement and body position), leading to improved balance and coordination.

II. Mental Benefits:

Stress Reduction:

Like traditional yoga, Chair Yoga incorporates breathing exercises and mindfulness techniques that help reduce stress and promote relaxation. By focusing on the breath and moving mindfully, participants can calm their minds, lower stress levels, and experience a sense of peace and tranquility.

Enhanced Cognitive Function:

Engaging in Chair Yoga can also benefit cognitive health. The combination of physical movement, breath control, and mindfulness helps stimulate brain function. Studies have shown that yoga practices, including Chair Yoga, can improve attention, memory, and executive function, which are critical for maintaining cognitive health as we age.

III. Emotional Benefits:

Increased Confidence:

Participating in Chair Yoga can boost self-confidence by providing seniors with a sense of accomplishment and capability. As they see improvements in their flexibility, strength, and balance, their confidence in their physical abilities grows, which can positively impact their overall quality of life.

Social Interaction:

Chair Yoga classes often provide a social setting where seniors can connect with others. This social interaction is crucial for emotional well-being, reducing feelings of loneliness and isolation. Being part of a group and sharing experiences can foster a sense of community and belonging.

GETTING STARTED

A. Safety First:

I. Precautions and Considerations for Practicing Chair Yoga:

Before embarking on your chair yoga journey, it's essential to consider certain precautions to ensure a safe and enjoyable experience. Chair yoga, though gentle and accessible, still involves physical activity, which requires mindful preparation.

1. Listen to Your Body: Pay attention to how your body feels during each movement. If you experience pain or discomfort, stop and modify the exercise. Remember, yoga is about gentle progress, not pushing through pain.

2. Stay Hydrated: Keep a bottle of water nearby and take sips as needed. Staying hydrated is crucial, especially if you're engaging in any form of physical activity.

3. Warm-Up and Cool Down: Start with gentle warm-up exercises to prepare your muscles and joints. Similarly, end your session with a cool-down period to help your body relax and recover.

4. Avoid Heavy Meals Before Practicing: It's best to practice yoga on an empty stomach or at least two hours after a meal. This helps avoid discomfort and enhances your ability to move freely.

II. Importance of Consulting with Healthcare Providers:

Before beginning any new exercise regimen, especially if you have existing health conditions, it's critical to consult with your healthcare provider. They can provide personalized advice based on your medical history and current health status.

1. Medical Clearance: Ensure you have clearance from your doctor, especially if you have conditions such as arthritis,

osteoporosis, heart disease, or respiratory issues.

2. Discuss Limitations: Talk about any physical limitations you might have. Your healthcare provider can advise which movements to avoid and suggest modifications.

3. Medication Awareness: Some medications may affect your balance or energy levels. Understanding these effects can help you practice more safely.

By taking these precautions and consulting with your healthcare provider, you lay a solid foundation for a safe and effective chair yoga practice.

B. Choosing the Right Chair:

I. Features of an Ideal Chair for Yoga:

The chair you use for chair yoga is more than just a seat; it's a vital piece of equipment that can significantly impact your practice. Here are the key features to look for:

1. Stability: Your chair should be sturdy and not easily tip over. Avoid chairs with wheels or swivel bases. A stable chair ensures your safety and confidence as you move.

2. Height: The chair should allow your feet to rest flat on the floor with your knees at a 90-degree angle. This helps maintain proper posture and balance during exercises.

3. Back Support: Look for a chair with a supportive backrest to help you maintain an upright position, especially during seated poses. A chair with a straight back is preferable over one with a reclined or contoured back.

II. Examples of Suitable Chairs:

Here are a few types of chairs that work well for chair yoga:

1. Dining Chairs: Sturdy dining chairs with straight backs and no armrests are often ideal. They provide good support and ample space for movement.

2. Folding Chairs: Metal or wooden folding chairs can be excellent choices, provided they are stable and offer good support. Ensure they lock securely when open.

3. Office Chairs: Simple office chairs without wheels or swivels can work, especially those with firm seats and backs. Adjustable height features can help you find the perfect fit.

C. Setting Up Your Space:

I. Creating a Calm and Safe Environment:

The environment where you practice chair yoga can significantly influence your experience. Here's how to create an ideal space:

1. Quiet Area: Choose a space away from noise and distractions. A quiet environment helps you focus and enhances the relaxation benefits of yoga.

2. Sufficient Space: Ensure there is enough room around your chair to move freely without bumping into furniture or walls. This helps prevent accidents and provides a sense of freedom.

3. Soft Lighting: Gentle, natural lighting is best. If this isn't possible, use soft, indirect lighting to create a calming atmosphere.

4. Ventilation: Make sure the space is well-ventilated. Fresh air can invigorate your practice and enhance your breathing exercises.

II. Necessary Equipment:

While chair yoga primarily requires just you and your chair, a few additional items can enhance your practice:

1. Yoga Mat: Place a yoga mat under your chair to prevent slipping and provide a stable surface for standing poses. It also adds comfort if you choose to do floor exercises.

2. Blocks and Straps: Yoga blocks can help with stability and bringing the floor closer to you in certain poses. Straps can aid in flexibility exercises, allowing you to extend your reach gently.

3. Comfortable Clothing:ABear loose, comfortable clothing that allows for full range of motion. Avoid tight or restrictive garments.

4. Small Towel: Keep a small towel nearby to wipe away any sweat and to provide additional support if needed.

By carefully considering these elements and setting up your space thoughtfully, you can create a comfortable, safe, and inviting environment for your chair yoga practice. With the right precautions, chair, and setup, you're well on your way to enjoying the many benefits of chair yoga for seniors.

BASIC CHAIR YOGA POSES

Chair Yoga for seniors is an empowering practice that adapts traditional yoga poses to be performed with the support of a chair. This chapter introduces you to basic chair yoga poses, designed to improve flexibility, strength, and balance. We will start with gentle warm-up exercises, followed by seated poses, and conclude with standing poses using the chair for support.

A. Warm-Up Exercises:

Before diving into the chair yoga poses, it's essential to prepare your body with gentle stretches. These warm-up exercises help to increase blood flow to your muscles, reduce stiffness, and prevent injuries. Here are a few simple warm-up exercises to get you started:

1. Neck Rolls:

Sit comfortably on your chair with your feet flat on the floor.

Slowly drop your chin to your chest, feeling a gentle stretch in the back of your neck.

Gently roll your head to the right, bringing your right ear towards your right shoulder.

Continue rolling your head back, looking up slightly, then to the left, and finally bringing your chin back to your chest.

Repeat this motion in a slow, controlled manner for 5-6 rotations in each direction.

2. Shoulder Shrugs:

Sit tall with your back straight and feet flat on the floor.

Inhale deeply and lift your shoulders up towards your ears.

Hold the position for a moment, then exhale and release your shoulders back down.

Repeat this movement 8-10 times, feeling the tension release from your shoulders.

3. Arm Circles:

Extend your arms out to the sides at shoulder height.

Begin to make small circles with your arms, gradually increasing the size of the circles.

After 10-15 seconds, reverse the direction of the circles.

Continue for another 10-15 seconds, then relax your arms by your sides.

4. Ankle Rolls:

Sit comfortably with your feet flat on the floor.

Lift your right foot off the ground and slowly rotate your ankle in a circular motion.

Complete 10 circles in one direction, then reverse and complete 10 circles in the opposite direction.

Repeat with your left foot.

These gentle warm-ups should leave you feeling relaxed and ready to move into the chair yoga poses.

B. Seated Poses:

Seated poses are performed while sitting on a chair, making them accessible and safe for seniors. These poses focus on improving posture, flexibility, and spinal health.

1. Seated Mountain Pose (Seated Tadasana)

Sit upright with your feet flat on the floor and your hands resting on your thighs.

Lengthen your spine, lifting through the crown of your head.

Roll your shoulders back and down, allowing your chest to open.

Engage your core and hold the pose for several breaths, feeling the stability and strength in your seated position.

2. Seated Cat-Cow Pose (Seated Marjaryasana-Bitilasana)

Sit towards the edge of the chair with your feet hip-width apart and hands on your knees.

Inhale and arch your back, lifting your chest and looking up (Cow Pose).

Exhale and round your spine, tucking your chin to your chest and drawing your belly in (Cat Pose).

Continue to flow between Cat and Cow poses with your breath for 8-10 cycles.

3. Seated Forward Bend (Seated Uttanasana)

Sit at the edge of your chair with your feet hip-width apart.

Inhale and lengthen your spine, then exhale and hinge forward from your hips, reaching your hands towards your feet.

Allow your head and neck to relax, feeling a gentle stretch in your back and hamstrings.

Hold the position for several breaths, then slowly rise back up to a seated position on an inhale.

C. Standing Poses with Chair Support:

Standing poses with chair support offer a great way to work on balance and strength while having the security of the chair for stability. These poses can be very beneficial for seniors looking to improve their overall physical health.

1. Chair-Assisted Warrior (Warrior II Variation)

Stand beside the chair, holding onto the backrest with your left hand.

Step your right foot back, keeping your left foot pointing forward and your right foot turned slightly out.

Bend your left knee, ensuring it is directly over your ankle, and extend your right leg straight.

Raise your right arm to shoulder height, reaching towards the back, while your left arm reaches forward.

Gaze over your left hand and hold the pose for several breaths.

Switch sides and repeat the pose on the opposite side.

2. Chair-Assisted Tree Pose (Vrksasana)

Stand beside the chair, using your left hand to hold onto the backrest for support.

Shift your weight onto your left foot and place the sole of your right foot against your left ankle or calf (avoid the knee).

Bring your palms together at your chest in a prayer position or keep one hand on the chair for balance.

Find a focal point to help maintain your balance and hold the pose for several breaths.

Switch sides and repeat the pose on the opposite side.

These basic chair yoga poses provide a gentle yet effective way to incorporate yoga into your daily routine. Practicing regularly can help enhance your physical and mental well-being, making everyday activities more enjoyable and less challenging. Remember to listen to your body and modify the poses as needed to suit your comfort and abilities.

CHAIR YOGA SEQUENCES

A. Daily Routine for Beginners:

Starting your day with a simple and gentle chair yoga routine can set a positive tone for the rest of the day. This sequence is designed to wake up your body, stretch your muscles, and energize you without overwhelming your system.

I. Simple Sequence to Start the Day:

1. Seated Mountain Pose (Tadasana)

Sit up straight with your feet flat on the ground.

Place your hands on your thighs, palms facing down.

Take a deep breath in, lengthening your spine, and relax your shoulders.

Hold for 5 breaths.

2. Neck Stretches

Slowly tilt your head to the right, bringing your right ear towards your right shoulder.

Hold for 3 breaths, feeling the stretch along the left side of your neck.

Repeat on the left side.

3. Seated Cat-Cow Stretch

Place your hands on your knees.

Inhale, arching your back and looking up (Cow Pose).

Exhale, rounding your back and tucking your chin to your chest (Cat Pose).

Repeat for 5 breaths.

4. Seated Forward Bend (Uttanasana)

Inhale, raising your arms overhead.

Exhale, hinge forward from your hips, reaching your hands towards your feet.

Hold for 5 breaths, feeling a gentle stretch in your back and hamstrings.

5. Seated Side Stretch

Raise your right arm overhead, leaning slightly to the left.

Hold for 3 breaths.

Repeat on the other side.

6. Seated Spinal Twist

Place your right hand on the back of the chair and your left hand on your right knee.

Inhale, lengthen your spine.

Exhale, twist to the right.

Hold for 3 breaths, then switch sides.

B. Balance and Stability Sequence:

Maintaining balance and stability is crucial as we age. This sequence focuses on poses that help improve your balance and enhance your stability, all while using the chair for support.

I. Focus on Poses that Improve Balance:

1. Seated Marching

Sit up straight with your feet flat on the ground.

Lift your right foot a few inches off the ground, then lower it.

Repeat with your left foot.

Continue marching for 1-2 minutes.

2. Seated Leg Lifts

Sit at the edge of your chair.

Extend your right leg out straight, then lower it back down.

Repeat with your left leg.

Do 10 lifts on each side.

3. Chair Stand:

Sit at the edge of your chair with your feet hip-width apart.

Place your hands on your thighs or use the armrests for support.

Lean forward slightly and press through your feet to stand up.

Slowly sit back down.

Repeat 5-10 times.

4. Heel Raises

Sit with your feet flat on the ground.

Lift your heels off the ground, coming onto the balls of your feet.

Lower your heels back down.

Repeat 10-15 times.

5. Seated Tree Pose

Sit up straight with your feet flat on the ground.

Place your right foot on the inside of your left ankle or shin.

Bring your hands to your heart or raise them overhead.

Hold for 3-5 breaths, then switch sides.

C. Strength and Flexibility Sequence:

Building muscle strength and increasing flexibility are essential for maintaining independence and preventing injuries. This sequence includes poses that focus on both aspects.

I. Poses that Build Muscle Strength and Increase Flexibility

1. Seated Warrior I (Virabhadrasana I)

Sit sideways on the chair with your right side facing the chair back.

Extend your right leg behind you, keeping your left knee bent.

Raise your arms overhead.

Hold for 5 breaths, then switch sides.

2. Seated Warrior II (Virabhadrasana II)

Sit sideways on the chair with your right side facing the chair back.

Extend your right leg behind you and your left leg in front, forming a 90-degree angle with your knee.

Extend your arms out to the sides at shoulder height.

Hold for 5 breaths, then switch sides.

3. Seated Hamstring Stretch:

Sit at the edge of your chair.

Extend your right leg out in front of you, heel on the ground, toes pointing up.

Hinge forward at your hips, reaching towards your toes.

Hold for 5 breaths, then switch sides.

4. Seated Knee Lifts:

Sit up straight with your feet flat on the ground.

Lift your right knee towards your chest, holding it with your hands.

Hold for 3 breaths, then lower.

Repeat with your left knee.

5. Seated Figure Four Stretch:

Sit with your feet flat on the ground.

Place your right ankle on your left knee.

Gently press down on your right knee, feeling a stretch in your right hip.

Hold for 5 breaths, then switch sides.

D. Relaxation and Stress Relief Sequence:

Relaxation and stress relief are vital for overall well-being. This sequence includes calming poses and breathing exercises to help you unwind and release tension.

I. Calming Poses and Breathing Exercises:

1. Seated Forward Bend with Relaxation

Sit at the edge of your chair with your feet flat on the ground.

Hinge forward from your hips, resting your torso on your thighs.

Let your arms hang down towards the ground.

Hold for 5-10 breaths.

2. Seated Child's Pose (Balasana)

Sit back in your chair with your feet flat on the ground.

Hinge forward from your hips, resting your torso on your thighs.

Rest your forehead on your knees and let your arms hang down.

Hold for 5-10 breaths.

3. Seated Shoulder Rolls

Sit up straight with your feet flat on the ground.

Roll your shoulders up towards your ears, then back and down.

Repeat 5 times in each direction.

4. Seated Belly Breathing

Sit comfortably with your feet flat on the ground.

Place one hand on your belly and the other on your chest.

Inhale deeply through your nose, allowing your belly to rise.

Exhale slowly through your mouth, letting your belly fall.

Continue for 5-10 breaths.

5. Seated Meditation

Sit comfortably with your feet flat on the ground and your hands resting on your thighs.

Close your eyes and take a few deep breaths.

Focus on your breath, letting go of any tension or stress.

Stay in this meditative state for 5-10 minutes, or as long as you like.

By incorporating these chair yoga sequences into your daily routine, you can improve your overall physical and mental well-being. Remember to listen to your body and adjust the poses as needed to ensure a safe and enjoyable practice.

BREATHING TECHNIQUES AND MEDITATION

A. Importance of Breath in Yoga:

Breath is the cornerstone of any yoga practice. For seniors, mastering the art of breathing not only enhances the physical benefits of yoga but also nurtures mental and emotional well-being. Understanding and controlling your breath can transform your yoga practice from a mere physical exercise into a holistic experience that balances body, mind, and spirit.

I. How Breath Control Enhances Yoga Practice:

In yoga, breath is referred to as "prana," which means life force. By consciously controlling your breath, you can direct this life force throughout your body, promoting relaxation and focus. Here's how breath control can enhance your yoga practice:

1. Increases Oxygen Flow: Deep, controlled breathing increases the intake of oxygen, nourishing your muscles and organs, and enhancing overall vitality.

2. Reduces Stress and Anxiety: Slow, deliberate breathing activates the parasympathetic nervous system, which calms the mind and reduces stress hormones.

3. Improves Concentration: Focusing on your breath anchors your mind, preventing it from wandering and enhancing your ability to stay present during your practice.

4. Enhances Flexibility and Strength: Coordinating breath with movement helps synchronize the body's natural rhythms, making poses feel more fluid and natural.

5. Promotes Detoxification: Deep breathing helps expel toxins from the body through the lungs, supporting overall health.

Incorporating breath control into your chair yoga routine ensures that you maximize these benefits, making each session more effective and enjoyable.

B. Basic Breathing Techniques:

Mastering basic breathing techniques is the first step toward a more fulfilling yoga practice. Here, we'll explore two fundamental techniques: diaphragmatic breathing and alternate nostril breathing.

I. Instructions for Diaphragmatic Breathing:

Diaphragmatic breathing, also known as belly breathing, involves using your diaphragm to take deep breaths, which maximizes oxygen intake and promotes relaxation.

Instructions:

1. Sit Comfortably: Sit upright in your chair with your feet flat on the floor. Place your hands on your abdomen.

2. Inhale Deeply: Take a slow, deep breath in through your nose, allowing your abdomen to expand as your diaphragm moves downward. Feel your belly rise under your hands.

3. Exhale Slowly: Exhale gently through your mouth, allowing your abdomen to fall as your diaphragm moves upward. Feel your belly contract.

4. Focus on Your Breath: Repeat this process, focusing on the rise and fall of your abdomen. Aim for a count of four on the inhale and four on the exhale, gradually increasing the duration as you become more comfortable.

II. Instructions for Alternate Nostril Breathing:

Alternate nostril breathing, or Nadi Shodhana, balances the left and right hemispheres of the brain, promoting mental clarity and calm.

Instructions:

1. Sit Comfortably: Sit upright in your chair with your feet flat on the floor. Use your right thumb to close your right nostril.

2. Inhale Through the Left Nostril: Take a slow, deep breath in through your left nostril.

3. Switch Sides: Close your left nostril with your right ring finger and release your right nostril. Exhale slowly through your right nostril.

4. Inhale Through the Right Nostril: Inhale deeply through your right nostril.

5. Switch Sides Again: Close your right nostril with your right thumb, release your left

nostril, and exhale slowly through your left nostril.

Repeat this process for several minutes, focusing on your breath and the sensation of air moving through your nostrils. This technique helps to balance your energy and clear your mind.

C. Introduction to Meditation:

Meditation is a powerful tool for calming the mind and enhancing mental clarity. For seniors, incorporating simple meditation practices into your routine can improve focus, reduce stress, and promote a sense of peace and well-being.

I. Simple Meditation Practices to Calm the Mind:

Here are a few straightforward meditation techniques that you can practice alongside your chair yoga:

1. Mindful Breathing:

Sit comfortably with your eyes closed.

Focus on your breath as you inhale and exhale.

Notice the sensation of air entering and leaving your body.

If your mind wanders, gently bring your focus back to your breath.

Continue this practice for 5-10 minutes.

2. Body Scan Meditation:

Sit comfortably with your eyes closed.

Take a few deep breaths to relax. Begin by focusing on your toes, noticing any sensations.

Slowly move your attention up through your body – feet, legs, hips, torso, arms, neck, and head.

Spend a few moments focusing on each part, releasing tension as you go.

Finish with a few deep breaths and a sense of overall relaxation.

3. Visualization:

Sit comfortably with your eyes closed.

Take a few deep breaths to relax.

Visualize a peaceful place, such as a beach, garden, or forest.

Imagine yourself in this place, noticing the sights, sounds, and smells.

Spend a few minutes immersing yourself in this tranquil setting.

Gradually bring your focus back to the present moment, feeling refreshed.

Incorporating these meditation practices into your daily routine can greatly enhance your overall sense of well-being, making your chair yoga practice a truly holistic experience.

By understanding the importance of breath and integrating basic breathing techniques and meditation into your chair yoga routine, you can create a powerful practice that supports your physical, mental, and emotional health. Remember, the key is consistency and mindfulness – making each breath and each moment count.

MODIFICATIONS AND ADAPTATIONS

Chair yoga is a gentle form of yoga that is practiced while sitting in a chair or using a chair for support. This makes it an excellent option for seniors, particularly those with limited mobility or specific health conditions. In this chapter, we'll explore how to adapt yoga poses to meet individual needs and how to use various props to provide additional support and enhance the practice.

Adapting Poses for Different Needs:

Chair yoga offers a range of adaptations to accommodate various physical abilities and health conditions. Whether you are dealing with arthritis, recovering from surgery, or simply experiencing the natural changes that come with aging, there are modifications that can make yoga both accessible and beneficial.

Variations for Individuals with Limited Mobility:

1. Seated Mountain Pose (Tadasana)

Standard Pose: Sit up tall in your chair with your feet flat on the floor, hip-width apart. Place your hands on your thighs or alongside your body, and lengthen your spine.

Adaptation: For those with limited mobility in the upper body, rest your hands on your thighs or on the armrests of the chair. Focus on lengthening through the spine and grounding through your feet.

2. Seated Forward Bend (Paschimottanasana)

Standard Pose: Sit on the edge of the chair, extend your legs straight in front of you with feet flexed, and gently bend forward from the hips, reaching toward your toes.

Adaptation: If extending the legs is challenging, keep your knees bent. Place your hands on your thighs or shins instead of reaching for your toes. Focus on the gentle stretch in your back and hamstrings.

3. Seated Cat-Cow Stretch (Marjaryasana-Bitilasana)

Standard Pose: Sit with your hands on your knees. On an inhale, arch your back and lift your chest and chin (Cow Pose). On an exhale, round your spine and tuck your chin toward your chest (Cat Pose).

Adaptation: If spinal movement is limited, perform smaller movements. Even slight flexing and extending of the spine can help maintain mobility and relieve tension.

Variations for Specific Health Conditions:

1. Osteoporosis

Avoid: Forward bends and poses that involve twisting of the spine.

Adaptation: Focus on gentle, supported backbends and poses that strengthen the spine and improve posture. Seated spinal twists should be done cautiously, avoiding deep twists.

2. Arthritis

Adaptation: Prioritize gentle movements and incorporate longer warm-up periods to ease joint stiffness. Use props for additional support and avoid poses that put pressure on sensitive joints.

3. Cardiovascular Conditions

Adaptation: Avoid poses that involve holding the breath or excessive exertion. Focus on gentle, flowing movements and incorporate restorative poses to promote relaxation.

Using Props for Support:

Props can be invaluable in making chair yoga more accessible and comfortable. They provide support, enhance stability, and allow for deeper relaxation. Here, we'll look at how to use yoga blocks, straps, and cushions effectively.

Yoga Blocks:

1. Seated Forward Bend (Paschimottanasana) with Blocks

Place a yoga block on each side of your feet. As you bend forward, rest your hands on the blocks instead of reaching for your toes. This provides support and reduces strain on your lower back.

2. Supported Bridge Pose (Setu Bandhasana)

Sit back in your chair and place a block under each foot to elevate your feet slightly. This modification can help alleviate discomfort in the lower back and hips.

Yoga Straps:

1. Seated Hamstring Stretch

Loop a yoga strap around the ball of one foot while extending the leg. Hold the ends of the strap and gently pull to deepen the stretch. This is especially useful for those with limited flexibility.

2. Seated Shoulder Stretch

Hold a strap in both hands behind your back, keeping your arms extended. Lift the strap slowly to stretch your shoulders and chest, maintaining a comfortable range of motion.

Cushions and Bolsters:

1. Seated Meditation

Place a cushion or bolster on your chair seat to provide extra padding and elevate your hips. This can help reduce discomfort in the lower back and hips during seated meditation.

2. Seated Reclining Pose

Use a bolster or cushion to support your lower back as you lean back in your chair. This provides gentle support and helps maintain proper alignment.

Putting It All Together:

Adapting chair yoga poses and using props effectively can transform your practice, making it more accessible, enjoyable, and beneficial. Always listen to your body and adjust poses to suit your individual needs. Chair yoga is about creating a practice that feels right for you, promoting physical health, mental well-being, and a sense of empowerment.

In the next chapter, we will delve into a series of specific chair yoga sequences designed to target different areas of the body, offering a comprehensive approach to your yoga practice. Whether you're looking to improve flexibility, build strength, or simply find relaxation, these sequences will provide a structured path to achieving your goals.

OVERCOMING COMMON CHALLENGES

Embarking on a chair yoga journey as a senior can be immensely rewarding, but it often comes with its own set of challenges. Understanding and overcoming these challenges is key to ensuring a safe, enjoyable, and sustainable practice. This chapter will address three main areas: dealing with physical limitations, staying motivated, and listening to your body.

A. Addressing Physical Limitations:

As we age, physical limitations such as arthritis, joint pain, and reduced flexibility can become more prevalent. However, these should not deter you from practicing yoga. With the right strategies, you can adapt your practice to suit your body's needs and reap the benefits of chair yoga.

I. Strategies for Dealing with Arthritis, Joint Pain, and Other Common Issues:

1. Gentle Movements: When dealing with arthritis and joint pain, it's crucial to focus on gentle movements. Chair yoga allows you to perform poses with support, reducing the strain on your joints. Start with simple stretches that mobilize your joints without causing discomfort. For example, gentle wrist circles, shoulder rolls, and ankle rotations can help maintain joint flexibility.

2. Use of Props: Props such as cushions, blocks, and straps can make yoga poses more accessible. A cushion on your chair can provide additional support and comfort for your back and hips. Straps can assist in reaching your feet or hands when your range of motion is limited, allowing you to experience the benefits of a stretch without overexertion.

3. Modified Poses: Modifying poses to accommodate your limitations is a

fundamental aspect of chair yoga. For instance, if a standing pose like Warrior II is challenging, you can perform it while seated. Extend one leg to the side and reach your arms out parallel to the floor, maintaining the pose's essence while ensuring your safety.

4. Consistent Practice: Regular practice can significantly improve your flexibility and strength over time. Even a few minutes of daily chair yoga can make a difference. Consistency helps in reducing stiffness and maintaining joint health, making movement more comfortable.

5. Consult a Professional: If you have severe arthritis or other medical conditions, consult a healthcare professional or a certified yoga instructor who can guide you through personalized modifications and ensure you practice safely.

B. Staying Motivated:

Maintaining motivation for a regular yoga practice can be challenging, especially when starting something new. However, there are several strategies to help you stay committed and enjoy your chair yoga journey.

I. Tips for Maintaining a Regular Practice:

1. Set Realistic Goals: Start with small, achievable goals. Instead of committing to an hour-long session every day, begin with 10-15 minutes. Gradually increase the duration as you become more comfortable with your practice.

2. Create a Routine: Establishing a regular routine can help make yoga a habit. Choose a specific time of day that works best for you, whether it's in the morning to energize your day or in the evening to unwind.

3. Find a Support System: Practicing with a friend or joining a class can provide support and accountability. Sharing your progress and

challenges with others can keep you motivated and make the experience more enjoyable.

4. Track Your Progress: Keeping a journal of your yoga practice can be encouraging. Note how you feel before and after each session, any improvements in your flexibility or strength, and any challenges you encounter. Reflecting on your progress can boost your motivation.

5. Enjoy the Process: Focus on the enjoyment and relaxation that yoga brings rather than just the end goals. Celebrate the small victories and appreciate the time you spend caring for your body and mind.

C. Listening to Your Body:

One of the fundamental principles of yoga is to listen to your body. Understanding the difference between discomfort and pain is crucial to ensure you practice safely and effectively.

I. Understanding the Difference between Discomfort and Pain:

1. Discomfort vs. Pain: Discomfort in yoga often means you're stretching your limits, which can be a part of building flexibility and strength. It might feel like a gentle pulling or mild soreness after practice. Pain, however, is sharp, intense, and persistent. It signals that you may be pushing your body too far and could risk injury.

2. Respect Your Limits: It's important to respect your body's limits. If a pose feels painful, stop and adjust or rest. Pushing through pain can lead to injuries and setbacks. Chair yoga is about finding what works for you, not about achieving a specific pose.

3. Modify When Needed: Never hesitate to modify poses to suit your comfort level. Use props or ask for guidance if you're unsure how to adjust a pose. Your practice should be personalized to your needs and abilities.

4. Tune Into Your Breath: Your breath is a powerful tool in yoga. If you find your breath becoming strained or labored, it may indicate you're pushing too hard. Slow, deep, and steady breathing helps you stay within a safe and beneficial range of motion.

5. Post-Practice Reflection: After each session, take a moment to reflect on how your body feels. Notice any areas of tightness, discomfort, or relaxation. This reflection can help you understand what your body needs in future practices and ensure you're progressing safely.

By addressing physical limitations with mindful strategies, staying motivated with practical tips, and listening to your body's signals, you can overcome common challenges in your chair yoga practice. Embrace this journey with patience and self-compassion, and you'll find that the benefits extend far beyond the physical, enhancing your overall well-being.

INTEGRATING CHAIR YOGA INTO DAILY LIFE

Chair Yoga offers a gentle, accessible way for seniors to enhance their physical and mental well-being. This chapter focuses on incorporating Chair Yoga into daily life, ensuring it becomes a natural, enjoyable part of your routine.

A. Incorporating Yoga into Routine Activities:

I. Simple Stretches and Poses for Different Times of the Day:

Chair Yoga can be seamlessly integrated into your daily schedule, offering benefits at various times of the day. Here are some simple stretches and poses for different parts of your day:

Morning: Energize and Awaken

Start your day with gentle stretches to wake up your body and mind.

1. Seated Mountain Pose (Tadasana): Sit up straight with feet flat on the floor, hands resting on your thighs. Inhale deeply, lengthening your spine, and exhale slowly. This pose helps improve posture and breathing.

2. Seated Cat-Cow Stretch: Sit towards the edge of the chair with feet hip-width apart. On an inhale, arch your back and look up (Cow Pose). On an exhale, round your spine and tuck your chin to your chest (Cat Pose). Repeat 5-10 times to enhance spinal flexibility.

3. Seated Forward Bend (Uttanasana): Sit with feet hip-width apart, inhale to lengthen your spine, and exhale as you hinge at the hips, reaching your hands towards the floor. This stretches your back and hamstrings, preparing you for the day ahead.

After Meals: Aid Digestion and Relaxation:

Post-meal stretches can aid digestion and promote relaxation.

1. Seated Spinal Twist: Sit up straight with feet flat on the floor. Place your right hand on the back of the chair and your left hand on your right knee. Inhale, lengthen your spine, and exhale, gently twisting to the right. Hold for a few breaths and switch sides. This twist stimulates digestion and relieves tension.

2. Seated Side Stretch: Sit with feet flat on the floor. Inhale, lift your right arm overhead, and exhale, lean to the left, stretching the right side of your body. Hold for a few breaths and switch sides. This stretch helps with digestion and relieves bloating.

Before Bed: Unwind and Prepare for Rest

End your day with calming poses to unwind and prepare for a restful sleep.

1. Seated Forward Fold: Sit with feet flat on the floor, inhale to lengthen your spine, and exhale as you fold forward, resting your torso on your thighs and letting your head hang. This pose calms the nervous system and relieves tension.

2. Seated Neck Stretch: Sit up straight, inhale, and on an exhale, gently drop your right ear towards your right shoulder. Hold for a few breaths and switch sides. This stretch releases neck tension accumulated throughout the day.

3. Deep Breathing Exercise: Sit comfortably, close your eyes, and take slow, deep breaths. Inhale through your nose for a count of four, hold for a count of four, and exhale through your mouth for a count of four. Repeat for several minutes to promote relaxation and prepare for sleep.

B. Chair Yoga for Social Settings:

I. Practicing Yoga with Friends or in Group Settings:

Chair Yoga can be a wonderful social activity, fostering community and connection. Practicing with friends or in group settings can enhance motivation and enjoyment.

1. Yoga Classes: Join a local Chair Yoga class at a community center or senior center. These classes often provide a supportive environment where you can practice under the guidance of an experienced instructor and socialize with peers.

2. Yoga Clubs: Form a Chair Yoga club with friends or neighbors. Set regular times to meet and practice together, sharing tips and encouraging each other.

3. Virtual Classes: For those who prefer or need to stay at home, virtual Chair Yoga classes offer an excellent alternative. Many online platforms offer live or recorded

sessions that you can follow with friends via video calls.

4. Chair Yoga Parties: Host a Chair Yoga party. Invite friends over for a session, followed by a healthy meal or refreshments. This can be a fun and engaging way to incorporate wellness into social gatherings.

Practicing Chair Yoga in social settings not only improves physical health but also boosts mental and emotional well-being through social interaction and support.

C. Chair Yoga in Care Facilities:

I. Benefits and Implementation in Senior Living Communities:

Chair Yoga is particularly beneficial in care facilities, where it can be integrated into the daily routine of residents to enhance their quality of life.

1. Physical Benefits: Regular Chair Yoga practice improves flexibility, strength, balance, and circulation. It helps manage chronic conditions like arthritis and hypertension, reduces the risk of falls, and promotes overall physical health.

2. Mental and Emotional Benefits: Chair Yoga reduces stress, anxiety, and depression. It enhances mood, promotes relaxation, and fosters a sense of well-being. Group sessions can also alleviate feelings of loneliness and isolation.

3. Cognitive Benefits: The mindful aspect of yoga improves cognitive function, concentration, and memory. Breathing exercises and meditation can enhance mental clarity and reduce cognitive decline.

Implementation Strategies:

1. Regular Classes: Schedule regular Chair Yoga classes led by trained instructors. These

can be held in common areas or dedicated wellness rooms to ensure accessibility for all residents.

2. Staff Training: Train care facility staff in basic Chair Yoga techniques so they can lead informal sessions and encourage residents to practice daily.

3. Personalized Programs: Offer personalized Chair Yoga programs tailored to the individual needs and abilities of residents. This can include one-on-one sessions for those who may need extra assistance.

4. Integration into Daily Routine: Encourage residents to incorporate Chair Yoga into their daily routine by offering short sessions throughout the day, such as morning stretches, post-meal digestion aids, and evening relaxation exercises.

5. Community Involvement: Involve family members and volunteers in Chair Yoga

sessions. This creates a sense of community and support, enriching the experience for residents.

By integrating Chair Yoga into the daily life of seniors, whether at home, in social settings, or within care facilities, we can foster a healthier, more engaged, and happier community. The gentle, accessible nature of Chair Yoga makes it an ideal practice for seniors, promoting physical health, mental clarity, and emotional well-being.

PERSONAL STORIES AND TESTIMONIALS

In the serene corners of senior centers, community halls, and even within the comfort of their own homes, chair yoga has quietly transformed the lives of many older adults. This chapter delves into the intimate narratives of those who have embraced this gentle practice, as well as insights from experts who have witnessed its profound effects firsthand.

A. Success Stories:

I. Experiences of Seniors who have Benefited from Chair Yoga:

Amidst the soft hum of peaceful breathing and gentle stretching, lives are being enriched in ways both expected and surprising. Take Martha, for instance, a sprightly 75-year-old who had all but resigned herself to a sedentary lifestyle due to arthritis. "I thought yoga was for the flexible and young," Martha chuckles, her eyes twinkling with newfound vigor. "But then my granddaughter introduced me to chair yoga. It's like a gentle awakening for my joints. I move more freely now than I have in years!"

Martha's story is just one among many. Across the country, seniors are discovering renewed vitality through chair yoga. Whether it's alleviating chronic pain, improving balance, or simply finding a moment of calm amidst life's hustle, the benefits are as diverse as the individuals who practice. Each success story echoes a testament to resilience and the power of adaptation, proving that age is no barrier to personal transformation.

B. Expert Insights:

I. Contributions from Yoga Instructors and Healthcare Professionals:

Behind every successful chair yoga practice lies a network of dedicated instructors and healthcare professionals who champion its efficacy. Yoga instructor Emily Ramirez shares her perspective: "Chair yoga is a beautiful bridge between movement and mindfulness. It meets seniors where they are physically and offers accessible pathways to wellness." Emily's sentiment is echoed by Dr. Michael Chen, a geriatrician specializing in senior health. "The holistic approach of chair yoga addresses not just physical health but also mental and emotional well-being," Dr. Chen affirms. "I've seen firsthand how it reduces stress and enhances overall quality of life."

These expert insights underscore chair yoga's credibility as a therapeutic tool validated by both ancient wisdom and modern science. As more research highlights its benefits—from improving flexibility and cardiovascular health to boosting mood and cognitive function—the integration of chair yoga into senior wellness programs continues to grow. Through the collaborative efforts of instructors, healthcare providers, and enthusiastic participants, chair yoga stands as a beacon of hope and healing for seniors everywhere.

CONCLUSION

In concluding our journey through the practice of chair yoga for seniors, it is essential to reflect on the transformative potential and enduring benefits that this gentle yet powerful form of yoga offers. Throughout this book, we have explored various poses, breathing techniques, and mindfulness practices tailored specifically to enhance the physical, mental, and emotional well-being of older adults.

A. Recap of Key Points:

Chair yoga provides a holistic approach to wellness by promoting flexibility, strength, balance, and relaxation—all crucial aspects of healthy aging. By adapting traditional yoga postures to the seated position, it ensures accessibility and safety, making it suitable for individuals of all abilities. Beyond the physical benefits, chair yoga fosters mental clarity, emotional stability, and a deep sense of inner calm. It encourages seniors to connect mindfully with their bodies, promoting a harmonious balance between physical health and mental peace.

The importance of chair yoga lies not only in its immediate effects but also in its long-term impact on overall health. Regular practice can alleviate joint stiffness, improve circulation, boost immune function, and reduce stress levels. Moreover, it cultivates a positive outlook and resilience, empowering seniors to embrace life with vitality and enthusiasm.

B. Encouragement for Continuous Practice:

As we conclude, I invite you to consider chair yoga not merely as an exercise routine but as a lifelong companion on your journey to health and well-being. Remember, every session is an opportunity to nurture yourself—body, mind, and spirit.

I encourage you to embrace chair yoga as a daily ritual, dedicating a few moments each day to reconnect with yourself and restore balance. Let each breath be a reminder of your inner strength and resilience. Celebrate every small progress and cherish the sense of accomplishment that comes with each practice session.

Above all, remain curious and compassionate toward yourself. Your journey with chair yoga is unique, and there is no destination—only a continuous exploration of your own potential for growth and vitality. Trust in the process, and let chair yoga be your guide to living fully and gracefully at every stage of life.

In conclusion, I extend my heartfelt gratitude for embarking on this journey with me. May chair yoga continue to enrich your life, bringing you health, joy, and a profound sense of well-being. As you integrate its teachings into your daily life, may you find peace in the present moment and strength in your inner resilience?

THE END

www.ingramcontent.com/pod-product-compliance
Lightning Source LLC
Chambersburg PA
CBHW052337220526
45472CB00001B/470